HEALTHY ON THE CAMPUS

Boost Your Immune System During The Rigors Of College

By Dr. Kathryn A. Boling MD

I hope that reading this book will provide you with solid strategies to improve your health, boost your immune system, and enhance your quality of life as you put in the time and the effort to excel in your college education.

Published by Dr. Kathryn A. Boling, Baltimore MD

Printed in the United States of America.

ISBN-13: 978-0692809891

Additional copies are available at special quantity discounts for bulk purchases for sales promotions, premiums, fundraising, and educational use.

For more information, please contact: Dr. Kathryn A. Boling, DrKathrynBoling@gmail.com

Table of Contents

Healthy on the Campus

For probably the first time in your life you will live away from your family. It is exciting to be on your own. You alone will make the decisions about how you will live your life. This book is a resource to help you stay safe and healthy during your time away at college. You may never need some of this information, but if you do, something you read here may even save your life or the life of a friend. At the very least, it is information that will help you stay healthy and feel good during this next phase of your education.

Rigors of College

College life, while not-quite real life is not-quite high school either. Classes are much more demanding which may lead to frequent late-night studying. That coupled with a college social life and the stress of adjusting to a new environment can seriously threaten your immune system. The good news is at your age, the immune system is normally quite robust. The bad news is that many things about college life negatively impact even the healthiest immune system.

Factors That Impair Your Immune System

- Stress: Unfortunately stress is a constant in college life. There is social stress: meeting new people, missing old people, figuring out exactly where you fit into the college milieu. There is physical stress: early classes, all-night studying for exams and late-night partying with friends. Persistently high stress levels can cause excessive levels of circulating cortisol, a steroid made in the adrenal gland. High levels of cortisol depress the immune system, making it harder to stay healthy.
- Poor diet: Unfortunately the typical college diet is high in fat and sugar. The saying "freshman fifteen" refers to the weight a freshman might gain from consuming this diet. But besides weight gain, eating a lot of sugar also depresses the immune system. The typical college diet interferes with the body's ability to fight off bacteria and viruses.
- Depression: Untreated depression can harm the immune system. In a Harvard Study of college students, 39 percent reported that they sought some form of mental health care during their time in school. Leaving family and friends is

hard, and it is not unusual to feel depressed sometimes – especially during the first several months of freshman year.

- Social disconnection hurts the immune system. Researchers have found that people who reported being lonely had more herpes infections (cold sores on their lips) than people reporting healthy relationships with family and friends. In fact, people who are isolated heal slower, have more colds, and get sicker on average than those who have a supportive network. The issue in college is that most students start their freshman year knowing very few people, making this time a particularly vulnerable time. Many college students initially feel isolated and lonely.
- Excessive intake of alcohol damages the immune system. College is notorious for party life and drinking. In fact, a national study of college students reported than about 20 percent of college students meet the criteria for alcohol use disorder. Binge drinking, even now and then, damages the immune system.

- Lack of sleep has also been shown to damage the immune system. Typically college students keep late night hours and do not get enough sleep. Less than 6-7 hours a night has been shown to impair the immune response to vaccines, an indication of immune suppression.
- About 70% of college students report that they have tried cigarettes. Smoking cigarettes may be one of the most damaging things you can do to your immune system. There are over 7000 chemicals released when a cigarette burns. Many of them are known to cause cancer. Smoking not only causes cell damage and cancer, but it depresses the very immune system that could save your life. Smoking even "socially" causes a chronic level of stress as the body tries to fight off the damaging effects of cigarettes. Other chemicals like tar suppress the immune system further. When you quit smoking, over time the immune system can recover. Some think that they can escape the damaging consequences of smoking by vaping or using electronic cigarettes. The bad news is that initial studies show that vaping and electronic cigarettes may be worse for you than smoking cigarettes.

Factors That Boost Your Immune System

A strong immune system can help prevent illness as well as help you recover faster should you become infected. The following factors have been shown to improve immune function:

- Stress reducers: Relaxation and/or meditation.
- A healthy diet with several servings of fruits and vegetables as well as an adequate dietary intake of Omega 3 fatty acids. Omega -3 fatty acids can reduce inflammation. Some studies have also shown Omega 3s to be beneficial in boosting the immune response. Multivitamins may also boost the immune system, and can't hurt considering that few college students eat healthy every day.
- Adequate sleep: Getting enough sleep is important in maintaining a healthy immune system. Try to get at least 6 hours of sleep a night.
- Nurturing your relationships: Having a supportive social network can boost the immune system. In the initial weeks of college, stay in contact with family and e-mail

or talk to friends from high school who may be attending different colleges.

- Prevention: Most kids who attend college are up to date with their vaccines. It is normally a requirement to attend college and may include two meningitis vaccines and the tetanus vaccines. But don't forget the flu vaccine each year – it is usually available late September or early October.
- Maintain a healthy-body weight with diet and regular exercise. Evidence proves that obesity can have a negative impact on the immune system.
- Stop unhealthy behaviors: Do not smoke and, if you drink alcohol, drink in moderation (no more than one alcoholic drink per day for women and two per day for guys)
- Hygiene: Wash hands frequently when attending classes, out in public, or in crowded places during the cold and flu season. Many viruses are not only spread from infected persons coughing and sneezing around you, but are also spread object to hand and then hand to your own eyes or mouth. For instance, someone ill opens the door and then you touch the doorknob and rub your eye a few minutes

later. Within a week you are sick. Also, be mindful if you are ill. Turn your head or cover your mouth when coughing (even soft coughs can spread virus droplets). Try not to cough or sneeze over food that others will eat.

Strategies To Keep Your Immune System Healthy: Daily Vitamin Supplements

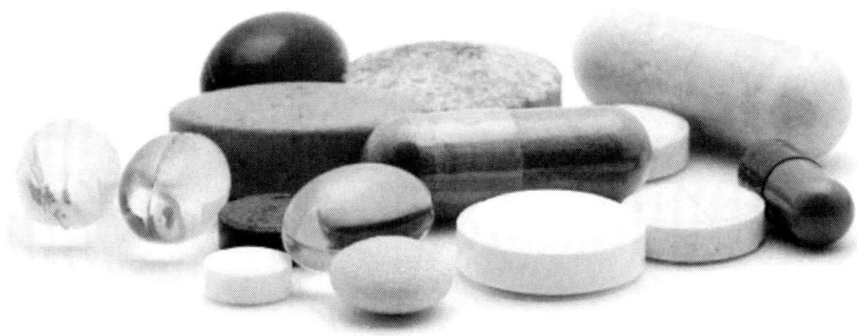

Even when you have a healthy diet, it is hard to absorb all the necessary nutrients to keep vitamin levels sufficient to boost your immune system. Most college students do not eat a healthy diet – college food is overwhelmingly unhealthy. The following are some supplements that you might consider taking.

- *Vitamin B12 1000mcg*: Vitamin B12 is good for your memory, can enhance your mood, give you energy and help with concentration and focus. It also strengthens your immune system. It can be taken either as a daily oral supplement or in an injection from your physician for a longer acting benefit.

- *Vitamin D 2000IU-10,000IU*: Vitamin D has many important functions including improving immune system function. People with normal vitamin D levels are less likely to get the flu and, more importantly in the long run, have decreased risk of heart disease and some cancers, including colon cancer. The farther north you reside or go to school, the more vitamin D you need to take (as your sun is further from the equator - and it is from the sun that we metabolize the majority of the vitamin D our bodies require). If you have a cold, temporarily increasing Vitamin D intake to a maximum of 20,000 IU daily may help you recover faster.
- *Vitamin C 500-1000mg*: Taking vitamin C regularly reduces the incidence and duration of colds.
- *Multivitamin with minerals*: Taking a multivitamin can compensate for deficits in the typical college diet and thus boost your immune system.
- *Probiotic*: A New Zealand study showed that people taking a daily probiotic had 40% fewer colds and fewer gastrointestinal illnesses. Choose an over-the-counter product that does not require refrigeration. I recommend

the probiotic Align™, available in virtually every grocery store or pharmacy.

- *Omega 3 Fish Oil*: This is a powerful anti-inflammatory supplement. Take 2000-3000mg daily. This can help with chronic inflammation (like sore post-game muscles if you play a sport) and ultimately lowers cortisol levels (the stress hormone). It is also great for your skin. If your brand of Omega 3 causes you to burp or taste fish later in the day, try freezing it and taking it frozen.
- *Magnesium 400mg:* Magnesium supplementation improves sleep and helps prevent leg cramps, keeps your bowels regular and relaxes the nervous system.

Supplements To Prevent The Common Cold

Colds cause a significant amount of discomfort including nasal discharge, sore throat, sinus stuffiness and cough. Most college students don't have time for a cold. Unfortunately there is no magic pill to cure the cold, but there are some herbal supplements that, when taken as recommended, can reduce your risk of catching a cold.

- *Astragalus 250-500mg (or as a tea) daily during cold and flu season (October through March):* A review from the Natural Medicine Comprehensive Database (NMCD) concluded there is evidence that taking astragalus long-term might help prevent colds. It may also be effective during allergy season to relieve symptoms of runny nose, itching and sneezing
- *Zink lozenges or syrup*: Studies show taking zinc reduces the average length of a cold in healthy people (by almost three days). Start zinc supplementation at the first sign of a cold as it works best if taken in the first 24 hours. Zinc may also prevent the common cold as well. I take zinc 50mg, Echinacea 100 - 300mg, and vitamin C

supplements 100 - 500mg daily during the cold and flu season. I believe it does prevent colds and this is backed up by a study that showed that zinc taken for five months reduced the incidence of colds in children. Airborne and Zycam also contain zinc (but do not taste very good) ***Never use any zinc nasal spray, it can permanently impair your sense of smell. Also do not take oral zinc year-round, as this may deplete copper in your system. Take breaks from zinc supplementation throughout the year.

- *Echinacea*: This herb increases the number of white blood cells, and these cells fight infection. Echinacea has been shown to prevent colds, but used alone its effect is small. Take 500mg three times daily if you have a cold, 300mg daily to prevent colds during the cold and flu season. You should be careful taking this if you have asthma, as it can worsen asthma symptoms. Check with your own physician before taking this if you have any underlying respiratory condition.

Cold And Flu Prevention And Treatment

Each year, about 20% of the US population will get the flu. Over two hundred thousand people will be hospitalized due to the severity of their illness and between 3,000 and 49,000 people will die from flu complications. With so many people working and living so close together in college, prevention of the flu before it strikes–and early treatment when it does–becomes paramount. The following strategies will lessen the impact from flu and colds:

- Get a yearly flu vaccine (especially if you have asthma, are a smoker or have any chronic respiratory illness). The Center for Disease Control recommends vaccination before the end of October each year.
- If you think you have the flu (severe body aches, fever, sore throat, respiratory symptoms, and sometimes nausea and/or vomiting) contact your physician as soon as possible. Certain medications can be prescribed to shorten the duration of the flu, but these medications must be started within the first 24-72 hours of symptoms in order to help you recover faster.

- Wash hands frequently or apply a hand sanitizer – especially during cold and flu season.
- Drink plenty of hydrating fluids. Remember, coffee, tea soda and alcohol are all dehydrating. I am not suggesting you forgo them completely. In fact, tea with lemon and honey can help alleviate sore throat. But I am recommending that you drink enough water to stay hydrated – at least 1½ glasses for every dehydrating drink plus a few more glasses on top of that during the day.
- Sleep with a humidifier. Viruses (flu and cold) replicate more effectively on dry mucus membrane. Moisturizing the air makes it harder for a virus to take hold and may reduce the duration and severity of your illness. Also, the moist air will help you feel better.
- Check with your own doctor, but in general for sinus pain and stuffiness, I recommend Sudafed™ (the kind you have to sign for at the pharmacy, not the kind on the shelf). I recommend taking 30mg twice daily with the last dose before 1 pm (this medication makes some people jittery and can interfere with sleep if taken too late in the day). Take this medication for three days. Also I

recommend buying Afrin™ 12 hour nasal spray and using this every 12 hours, but for no more than 48 hours. This medication can help you stay more comfortable during the very acute phase of your cold, but using it longer can result in something called rebound stuffiness. If you are flying home from school for breaks and you have a cold, take the Sudafed and 12 hour Afrin about 1 hour before your flight to prevent ear pain and ear injury on takeoff and landing. Do not take these medications if you have heart problems or high blood pressure without first checking with your doctor.

- Contact your doctor if symptoms last longer than 7-10 days as a secondary bacterial infection may have developed.
- Rest as much as possible (hard I know). Try to get at least 7 hours of sleep each night.

Personally, I use Alka-Seltzer Cold Plus™ (the original cherry flavored kind, not the kind that says nighttime or daytime. I don't like those formulas) once my severe symptoms have resolved and I am no longer using the Sudafed and the Afrin. I find that one packet at night keeps me pretty much symptom-free for about 24 hours without impacting my ability to work or study the next day.

Sleep Like A Baby

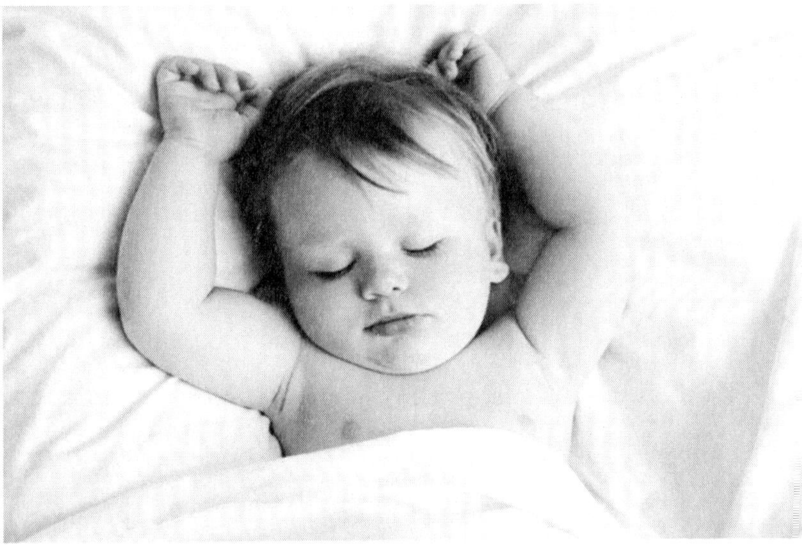

In college, hours are long and there is a lot of stress revolving around grades and testing. Because of this, many students have a difficult time unwinding at night. Then there is the complication of jet lag for those returning to school from home after a long weekend or school break. The following are herbal supplements than can help you get a good night's sleep and some that can help you adjust to the time changes that trigger jet lag.

- *Melatonin*: Melatonin is a hormone that our brains produce when the sun goes down. To help you fall asleep faster and perhaps sleep deeper and longer, take 1-3mg nightly about 30 minutes prior to bedtime. I recommend the brand from GNC as I know personally that this product works, and I have seen inconsistencies in other brands. Melatonin can help with jet lag as well if taken the first few nights after arriving from a different time zone.

- *Chamomile Tea*: Chamomile tea can relax you prior to bedtime as well as improve your daytime performance the following day.
- *Passionflower*: Passionflower tea or a 90mg tablet at night can calm anxiety and help with sleep. It may be especially beneficial for people who cannot "turn off their mind" at night.
- *Valerian Root*: Can be taken as an oral supplement of 300 to 600 mg or you can soak 2-3 grams (2000-3000mg) of dried herbal valerian root in one cup of hot water for 10 to 15 minutes. Drink the tea or take the supplement 30 minutes to two hours before bedtime. Valerian Root also helps with anxiety.

Aromatherapy

Certain odors have been proven to trigger a particular human response. Because of the olfactory response (our sense of smell), some odors will help calm us down, while others will increase alertness:

- *Lavender:* The smell of lavender relaxes you and can help you sleep. Putting some lavender oil on pillows or bed sheets can help you fall asleep faster and sleep deeper.
- *Jasmine:* The smell of Jasmine can be as calming as a sedative without the dangerous side effects.
- *Lemon*: The scent of lemon improves mood as well as cognitive function. When studying for a test, rub a bit of lemon scent on your wrists to ace the exam.
- *Peppermint:* Conversely, if you did not sleep well and find yourself groggy in the morning, sniffing some peppermint can help wake you up. I know of a few teachers who use the scent of peppermint in their classrooms during exams to help students focus.

Herbs to Avoid

Herbs are not necessarily benign, many are as potent as prescription drugs and their side effects can be just as dangerous. The following are herbs that were once recommended, but are now known to cause serious side effects and should be avoided.

- *Kava*: Once recommended as a sleep aid, this supplement can cause liver failure and may worsen depression. It is not safe to take this herb orally.
- *Comfry*: This herb is unsafe to take as it also can cause severe liver damage
- *Tryptophan*: It's ok to get your tryptophan naturally from that delicious Thanksgiving turkey or a cup of warm milk at night, but do not take this supplement as an oral capsule or pill as it has been linked to a disorder called EMS. EMS is a serious neurological condition with symptoms that include fatigue, intense muscle pain, nerve pain, swelling of the joints and damage to lungs, heart and liver.

Medication Help

Sometimes, in very severe cases, over-the-counter sleep aids – which are mostly antihistamines – may be necessary. However, do not take any sleep aids before discussing with your physician and do not drink alcohol with sleep aids. If over-the-counter medication fails to work, short-term prescription medication may be indicated. Again, discuss this with your doctor should you feel the need for prescription medication. Be aware that most prescription medications for sleep are Benzodiazepines or hypnotics and these medications may impair daytime performance and cause short-term memory loss – a bad side effect when you are trying to remember what you studied the previous night.

Sleep Hygiene

Besides using herbs, aromatherapy, and relaxation techniques to encourage better sleep, certain behaviors and strategies known as *sleep hygiene* can make a real impact on how fast you fall asleep, how restful that sleep is, and how long you remain asleep:

- A warm bath before bedtime may help you relax.

- Keep your bedroom at a comfortable temperature. Many people sleep better in a cooler room – try 68 degrees.
- Background white noise - like a fan or a sleep machine – may help you sleep better and reduce nighttime awakenings.
- Keep your bedroom dark.
- Avoid caffeine, nicotine and other stimulants several hours before bedtime.
- Do not use electronic devices the hour before sleeping – there is evidence the light from these devices can cause insomnia.
- Don’t exercise too late at night – the earlier you exercise the better as exercise tends to amp us up.
- Avoid a heavy meal or excessive snacking too close to bedtime. Also limit your intake of fluids 1-2 hours prior to bedtime.

Naps

Naps can be extremely beneficial. The length of your nap and the type of sleep you get helps determine the brain-boosting benefit.

A power nap of 10-20 minutes will allow you to wake up alert and ready to go. Short naps can boost your ability to learn a motor skill like playing an instrument.

Longer naps help boost memory and enhance creativity. Taking a 30-60 minute nap will help you with memorization (key when studying for a test).

A 60 to 90 minute nap can help you form new connections in the brain and solve creative problems.

Stress Reduction

Overall, reducing stress leads to a healthier immune system, decreased rates of illness, and increased psychological wellbeing. One or more of the following are good strategies to reduce stress:

- Aromatherapy can help relieve stress. Certain aromas (like lavender, jasmine and lemon) have been shown to reduce stress levels
- Listening to music and dancing (alone or with someone else) can reduce stress
- Laughter reduces the physical effects of stress (like fatigue) on the body
- Drinking black tea lowers cortisol levels and promotes relaxation
- Chewing gum can lower cortisol levels
- Getting a massage feels good and reduces stress.
- Talking about sex can actually lower blood pressure
- Getting or giving a hug is good for you - both emotionally and physically

- Spending time with an animal (especially a dog) can significantly improve your mood
- Keeping a journal of your feelings helps reduce stress
- Taking a walk (outside is best). Any form of exercise reduces stress
- Meditation might be one of the best stress reduction techniques of all

Sample Meditations

Muscle Relaxation

Lie in a comfortable position in bed or sitting in a chair and start with the head. Tense the muscles of the head to the count of 10 and then relax. Feel warmth in the relaxed muscles. Then tense the muscles in the neck and shoulders just as you did the head, followed by relaxation. Slowly move down the body tensing and relaxing the arms, chest, abdomen, legs, feet and toes. Once you have tensed and relaxed all the areas of the body, feel the warmth and relaxation begin again in your head and neck and allow it to stream downward through the same pathway in your body until you are warm from head to toes.

Breathing Meditation

Sit with your eyes partially or completely closed and turn your attention to your breathing. Breathe naturally, preferably in through your nose, out through your mouth and become aware of the feeling the air makes as it goes in and out, but do not try to control your breathing. Feeling the sensation of breathing is the object of this meditation.

The mind is very busy, and at first it may seem like it becomes even busier as you concentrate on the sensation. There is a temptation to follow the thoughts as they arise, but try to resist and go back to focusing on the sensation of just breathing in and out. Sometimes it helps to count the breaths to the number ten, starting over again at one. If you realize that the mind has wandered, simply refocus on breathing and start at the number where you left off. Do this meditation for as long as you desire.

Guided Meditation

Some people have trouble with breathing meditation. I am one of those people. But I have developed a kind of guided meditation that works for me; I will give you an example of it below. Of course, you are free to develop your own meditation or go online and download an audio file of a meditation that works well for you.

Take some deep breaths…. breathe deeply through your nose, hold your breath for a few seconds, then breath out through your mouth until you have a feeling of quietness. Breathe normally and imagine that you are standing at the top of a bluff looking down to a small inlet with a beach. It is calm and peaceful and you can hear the waves breaking gently at the water's edge below. Now start walking down the path to the beach. As you walk down, feel yourself becoming more and more relaxed. Feel your bare feet as they sink into the warm sand. Your path is winding, but every now and then you glimpse the sun glimmering off the water until you are on the beach. As you approach the edge of the water you notice that the instead of sand, the floor beneath the water is covered in tiny crystals; some are pink, some are blue and some are purple. There are many colors and each color imbues a specific power - you decide which powers go with which colors. For example, perhaps today you need wisdom and you have decided the pink crystals impart wisdom. If so, walk into the water and float above the pink crystals. Feel yourself becoming wiser as the power of the crystals engulfs your body. Or perhaps you need healing and you have decided the blue crystals have healing powers. If so, go to the blue crystals and feel the power as they slowly heal you of your physical or emotional pain. Whatever you need, there is a crystal color that can give you that exact thing. As you float above them and absorb the power of the crystals, relax even further. Breathe in and out, floating in the warm water, and feel the tension leave your body.

As I said above, you can make the crystals any color and give them any power you desire. Or you can create your own meditation, you are only limited by your own imagination. The important thing is to find something that works for you.

Boost Brain Power

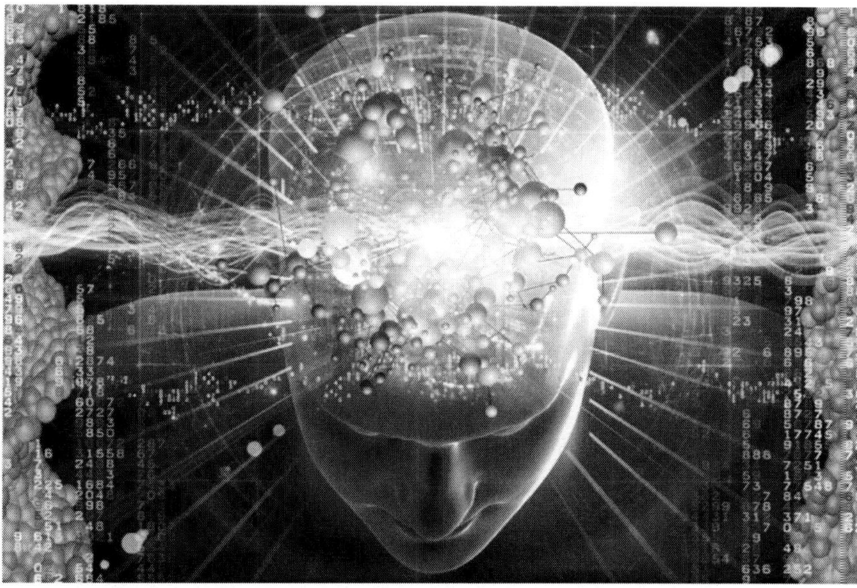

Keeping your brain healthy improves overall health. Many researchers and physician-scientists have been studying the brain and how it works. They have found some very interesting facts. Changing the way you eat may actually help your brain function more efficiently. Evidence indicates that diets high in salt, saturated fats and sugar actually shrink the brain over time, which is ironic considering the goals of a college education and the typical college diet. The following may help boost brain-power during some of the most challenging yeas of your life:

- DHA Omega 3 helps grow the brain – eat two servings of fish a week and take 1000mg of DHA daily (more if you can't commit to eating the fish)
- Flavonoids like green tea, quercetin (found in apple skins), beets, blueberries, caffeine (about 200mg daily), cocoa, pecans, red grapes, spinach, and tomatoes all improve blood flow to the brain.
- Vitamins your brain absolutely needs:
    - B12
    - Vitamin D
- Moderate alcohol intake is believed to protect brain and nervous system function – but moderate alcohol is no more than one drink a day for women and two a day for men.
- Meditation helps grow your brain
- Tai Chi, Yoga and Mindfulness grow the brain
- Changing your attitude with positive visualization and gratitude helps grow the brain – keep a gratitude diary
- Engaging emotionally with others helps improve brain function

- Memory exercises (just taking classes and studying for tests can enhance memory)
- Decrease stress and treat depression- both shrink your brain
- When I started medical school at age forty-nine, I was nervous that I might not be able to compete with the 22-24 year old minds of my classmates. I did some research and discovered a supplement that I feel has helped me boost my own brainpower. That supplement is phosphatidyl serine 300mg daily. For me, this not only supported memory, but also helped me maintain focus. If you decide to use this supplement yourself, make sure you are taking a plant-based product.

Drug and Alcohol Safety

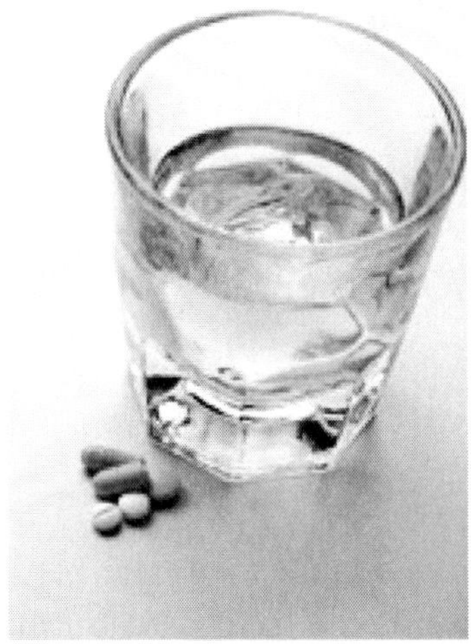

For some college students, college life has become synonymous with drinking alcohol. A Harvard study of graduating seniors found the following:

- *Nearly a quarter of the class said they drink more than twice a week.*
- *38 percent of students have tried marijuana, and 3 percent use it more than twice a week. Of marijuana users, 44 percent started in college; the rest started before college.*

- *Almost a quarter of the class used tobacco at least occasionally, with about 40 percent of users having started at college.*
- *16 percent of the class has tried at least one of the following: cocaine, ecstasy, mushrooms, LSD, or other illicit substances. Very large majorities of those who have used these drugs first tried them after starting college.*

You may not find these statistics alarming, but because of heavy drinking and experimental drug use, one in four college students report academic consequences that end up hurting them. These consequences include: missing class, falling behind in class, doing poorly on exams or papers, and lower grades overall. There are more serious consequences as well: suicide attempts, health problems, injuries, unsafe sex, and driving under the influence of alcohol, as well as vandalism, property damage, and involvement with the police.

Some college students never drink, and if that is you, the following will be of limited value. But for those who will drink, I am not advocating alcohol abstinence, as I do not believe that is realistic for most college students. What I am advocating is the following:

1. Talk to your parents before you leave for school about drinking. Know what your limits are – how much alcohol you can drink before you become impaired. Better to find this out at home with your parents than while out drinking with friends.

2. Think about ways to limit your drinking while out with friends. Sip your drinks to make them last longer. Try drinking one large glass of ice water for every alcoholic drink you consume. Not only does this slow down your alcohol intake, but it also helps prevent some of the symptoms of a hangover, as dehydration plays a big role in hangovers. Do not drink more than 3-4 alcohol beverages in any one sitting.

3. Eat food while you drink. In particular, try to eat foods that are higher in protein like beef, chicken and nuts. Avoid high fat foods as these foods can intensify alcohol absorption.

4. Appoint a designated driver or use Lyft™. I have a friend who is an attorney specializing in DUI cases. He has seen his case volume go down appreciably since Lyft™ came onto the scene. Take advantage and use Lyft™ or its local

equivalent to go from club to club or home after a night of partying.

5. Know what is in your drink. Some fruit-sweetened drinks contain a high percentage of alcohol or may have several types of alcohol in them, yet taste benign. It is easy to get extremely drunk on just one of these cocktails.

6. Avoid drinking alcohol on an empty stomach or on a very hot day when you are likely dehydrated. This can intensify feelings of intoxication.

7. Don't mix alcohol with other drugs, including over the counter medications like antihistamines or pain medications. Check with your physician regarding medication use and alcohol intake.

8. If you vomit, stop drinking immediately. Vomiting is the body's way of getting rid of toxins or poisons. Your body is telling you that you have had too much alcohol to drink so listen to it before you end up in the emergency room having your stomach pumped or worse.

9. Make a commitment to your friends and ask for one in return: if anyone becomes unresponsive you will take

them to the nearest emergency room or call 911. In the last ten years, hundreds of college students have died of alcohol poisoning. Many could have been saved had their friends recognized the severity of their symptoms and intervened.

10. If possible, have a designated sober friend to keep an eye on things – even if driving is not an issue.

Vaping Alcohol

The common use of e-cigarettes has also spawned the business of alcohol vaping - a process of inhaling a vaporized form of alcohol. Some have touted the benefit of getting the effects of drinking without the calories. But is it really a good alternative? Inhaling alcohol vapors has several potential health risks, including the most serious: the inability to determine exactly how much alcohol has been consumed and thus the risk of alcohol poisoning. When too much alcohol is consumed in the traditional manner, a protective mechanism kicks in and you vomit to expel alcohol from the stomach before it can be absorbed. When you vape alcohol, that protective mechanism is ineffective – making the possibility of alcohol poisoning and death even higher. But that is not the only negative. Vaping alcohol also causes irritation of the lungs and upper respiratory system, making you more vulnerable to respiratory infections and possibly more serious long-term respiratory consequences. There is even some preliminary research that indicates vaping alcohol may harm the brain in ways that can eventually lead to dementia.

STD prevention

Studies show that approximately 70% of students are virgins at the time of high school graduation, while only about 25% will graduate from college as virgins. That means out of every one hundred students, 45 will become sexually active during the college years. About 8% of college students report they have had 10 or more partners during their college years. Given that only 70% of sexually active adolescent men and a mere 58% of sexually active adolescent women report consistent condom use, STD and pregnancy prevention are important college topics.

STD prevention: The transmission of virtually all STDs (except some forms of HPV and in some unusual cases, herpes) can be prevented by the use of condoms. Sometimes patients tell me that they engage in intercourse, but their partner does not ejaculate inside them and, because of this, they think they are protected from pregnancy and STDs. The fact is, to effectively prevent STD transmission as well as prevent pregnancy, a condom needs to be on the penis whenever the penis is in the vagina - regardless of when or where ejaculation happens.

If you find yourself in a monogamous relationship and decide to forgo condom use, both partners should be tested and found to be negative for the following STDs before having sex without a condom: Gonorrhea, Chlamydia, HIV, Hepatitis B, Syphilis, and possibly Herpes.

1. **Chlamydia and Gonorrhea:** two of the most common STDs. A person can be infected with one or the other or both at the same time. These infections are transmitted through sexual contact. In a woman the bacteria lives in the cervix; in a man, the urethra. A person who has oral sex with an infected partner can even get a throat infection from these bacteria. Many women will not have symptoms, or if they do have symptoms they might be atypical – like urinary frequency or pelvic pain. In women, an untreated infection could cause infection in the fallopian tubes and ultimately lead to infertility. Men may have pain with urination and/or a discharge from the penis. You can be tested for these infections by a simple urine test or by direct culture. Antibiotics can be prescribed to cure these infections. To prevent infection in the first place, use condoms.

2. **HIV:** the most dreaded STD. It is transmitted by blood and body fluid like semen and vaginal secretions. Condoms, when used correctly, can reduce the risk of

contracting HIV. If you think you have been exposed to HIV by having unprotected sex with an HIV infected partner, you should seek medical attention immediately as you may be helped by something called PEP (post-exposure prophylaxis- antiviral HIV medications). PEP should be used only in emergency situations and must be started within 72 hours after an exposure to HIV. PEP treatment can be prescribed in cases of sexual assault by an HIV positive attacker or by someone with unknown HIV status. If you're prescribed PEP, you'll need to take it once or twice daily for 28 days. PEP reduces your risk of contracting HIV when administered in this manner, but it is not 100% effective.

3. **Herpes:** an STD that causes a lot of emotional angst, primarily because there is no cure. What many people do not completely understand is that a cold sore on your lip is caused by the herpes virus. This herpes virus is called Herpes Simplex Virus Type 1 (HSV 1). This is a common virus; about 80% of people have been exposed to this virus by adulthood. The virus can be transmitted to the genitalia of another person if oral sex happens during or right before an oral herpes outbreak. In that case the virus,

although now causing symptoms in the genitalia, would still be HSV Type 1.

Herpes Simplex Virus Type 2 is a different type of herpes infection that normally occurs on the genitalia. Once a person is exposed to and contracts herpes, they could suffer ongoing outbreaks. Some people are lucky enough to have only one outbreak and never have another outbreak again. Others might have several outbreaks every year. HSV Type 1 typically causes fewer outbreaks than HSV Type 2. In most cases, the first herpes outbreak is the worst. Symptoms can include a flu-like syndrome, fever, swollen glands, and painful blisters at the site of infection (usually the labia or anal area in a woman and the penis in the man). Symptoms can last from a few days to a couple of weeks in a severe outbreak. Anti-viral medication can be prescribed to shorten an outbreak as well as to suppress outbreaks in those unlucky enough to have multiple attacks.

Women who are pregnant and have a herpes outbreak at the time of delivery will need a cesarean section delivery to protect the newborn from exposure. Newborn babies can become very ill and even die if exposed to the herpes virus.

4. **Syphilis:** Syphilis is less common these days, but still a very serious STD. Syphilis develops in four different stages – each with its own set of symptoms. Initially, syphilis causes a sore called a chancre. Usually there is one sore at the site of infection, but some people may have several sores. Unlike herpes, which hurts a lot, the syphilis sore is usually painless and thus may be missed. It will heal on its own in about 6 weeks.

   The second stage of syphilis arises and a person may notice a non-itchy rash that starts of the trunk and eventually spreads all over the body including the hands and soles of the feet. At the same time there may be wart like sores in the mouth or the vagina, swollen glands, fever, sore throat and muscle aches. Symptoms can come and go and may last up to a year.

   The third stage, or latent stage, has no symptoms at all, and can last indefinitely. However, about 15% - 30% of people who progress to the latent stage of syphilis without treatment will go on to develop tertiary syphilis. With tertiary syphilis, the disease enters the brain and other parts of the body causing damage to the brain, nerves, eyes, heart, blood vessels, liver, bones and joints. In the earlier stages of syphilis, the disease can be easily treated with a Penicillin injection. Later in the disease, multiple doses of Penicillin may be needed. To protect yourself, use condoms when having sex and see your physician if you develop any of the above symptoms or fear you have been exposed.

5. **Hepatitis B:** Most college students have been vaccinated for Hepatitis B. Still, even with vaccination, a small percentage of vaccinated people do not develop immunity. Before college, you should have had your blood tested by your physician to make sure you are immune. Sometimes a Hepatitis B booster shot is needed. Again, condom use can protect you from exposure to Hepatitis B.

6. **HPV (Human Papillomavirus):** There are many types of HPV virus, most of them harmless. A type of HPV virus is responsible for common warts that infect many children and adults. HPV is so common that it is estimated that over the course of one's lifetime, virtually everyone will

come in contact with some sort of HPV virus because all that is needed to transmit the virus is skin-to-skin contact. Because of this, condoms are not as effective at preventing the spread of HPV as they are for say, Chlamydia or gonorrhea, so it is possible to get HPV even when using a condom correctly.

Relatively recently it was discovered that certain strains of HPV caused cervical cancer as well as some cancers of the throat and larynx. Now it is recommended that boys and girls at age 11-12 start the HPV vaccine series. Still, even if you have been vaccinated it is important for women to see their physician for pap smears once they reach the age of 21. Guidelines now recommend HPV testing (for the high risk cancer-causing types) once a woman reaches age 30. Currently there is no HPV testing available or recommended for men, but that may change in the future.

Firearm Threat

In 2015 there were 23 college campus shootings. The deadliest 2015 college shooting was at the Oregon's Umpqua Community College where ten people were killed and seven others were injured. The shooter was a fellow student. After entering the school and shooting a teacher in the head, the gunman ordered the rest of the class to get down on the ground. After they complied, he instructed those who were Christians to stand up. He then shot them one-by-one, even stopping to reload.

One student, who hid in a different classroom, told authorities that when she and her classmates heard the shooting they dropped to the floor and huddled behind backpacks and desks. Could any of them have done something different to save their lives? Possibly yes.

The first advice when confronted with a situation like the one described above is to stay calm, or at least as calm as possible. Panic in a life-threatening situation is completely understandable. The minute you become aware that you are panicking, you have to tell yourself to get focused and calm down. While this may sound impossible, I know it is not because I stopped myself from panicking while in a burning car after being hit by an 18-wheeler and it saved my life.

Staying calm allows you to think - of a way out, of a potential escape route, of a weakness the gunman might have and how you could exploit that weakness to your own advantage – anything that might give you an opportunity to stay safe and alive.

Second, the normal inclination of a group of people confronted by a gunman is to huddle together. Ironically that instinct to stay close to others is the worst thing you could do. Huddling together gives the gunman an easy target and keeps you all in the kill zone. Drifting apart or moving away from others actually makes it more difficult for the gunman to hit multiple people.

Third, as a last resort, when there is an active shooter in the building actually shooting and killing people, it is better to fight for your life than passively wait to die. For years we have told students to lock down and hide in their classrooms. One surviving student in Oregon reported to the following to authorities:

> *"...all of the students in my classroom dropped to the ground. They huddled together behind backpacks and chairs, underneath tables."*

Hiding behind a desk or a backpack will offer little protection if a shooter enters your room. Many reputable agencies, including homeland security, recommend that first and foremost, try to escape the area. If you are in an area far from the shooter, get out, even if others will not come with you. Leave your valuables and cell phones behind if you have to. Help others who might need your help to get away as well.

If you are unable to escape and in a visible area like a hallway, find a room where you can hide. Lock and barricade the door and **silence your cell phone**. The last thing you need is your phone ringing as the gunman looks for victims. Remain quiet, but be prepared to fight if the shooter enters the room. If there are several people in the room, make a plan. Place some of the stronger individuals off to the side of the door, positioned to surprise and take down the shooter should he enter. This is also in line with the following instructions by Homeland Security:

> *When the shooter is at close range and you cannot flee, your chance of survival is much greater if you try to incapacitate him/her.*

Safety for Women

In a survey of 24,000 college students a little over 10 percent reported an attempted rape. In the general population, 15 to 25% of women report that they have been attacked, molested, or raped. This makes safety tips for women in particular very timely and important. Safety tips for women in college can be found below:

1. Be aware of your surroundings. Too often, we are looking at our cell phones and texting while in unfamiliar places. As a woman, you must stay aware of your surroundings to protect yourself. Make eye contact with those around you. Many times an attacker will avoid a victim who appears confident or who has been looking at them directly as they fear the woman may later be able to identify them.

2. Listen to your intuition. My ex-husband, a police officer, told me many times that female victims often told him that they had an intuition or felt uncomfortable but did not act on their feelings because they were afraid of offending the perpetrator or looking silly. For instance, one woman was waiting for an elevator and when it opened she felt uncomfortable, but worried how she might appear if she

did not get in. She was attacked in that elevator. Her intuition was right, but she ignored it. If you find yourself feeling uncomfortable, listen to your intuition. It could save your life. If you are walking to your car and you think that someone walking nearby might try to hurt you: run to your car, get in and lock the door. It doesn't matter if you think you look silly or rude. What matters is staying safe.

3. Many experts including my ex-husband also give this advice: If someone attempts to abduct you, never leave the site of abduction even if the attacker has a knife or a gun. Women who allow an attacker to remove them from the original crime scene are 10 times more likely to be injured or killed. Better to be shot or stabbed in the parking lot of a mall than taken to a remote area where you can be tortured and killed.

4. If you are able, run! Experts say than an assailant with a gun will only hit you 4 out of 100 times if you run. Escape the area if possible.

5. If you are unable to run and you think you have a chance to get away by fighting - fight. Many experts recommend

self-defense courses for women. These courses should prepare you to defend yourself in close quarters. If you do fight, aim for your assailant's vulnerable areas: eyes, head (nose especially), groin and the instep of the foot.

6. Carry your car keys in your hand when you go to the car. This prevents fumbling to find the keys if you need to get into your car fast.

7. When you go out, go out with friends and do not split up. Groups of two or more are less likely to be accosted than a woman alone.

8. Make a pact with friends to keep an eye on each other. Have a code word that all of you know to use in any situation if one of you feels unsafe.

Unexpected Problems

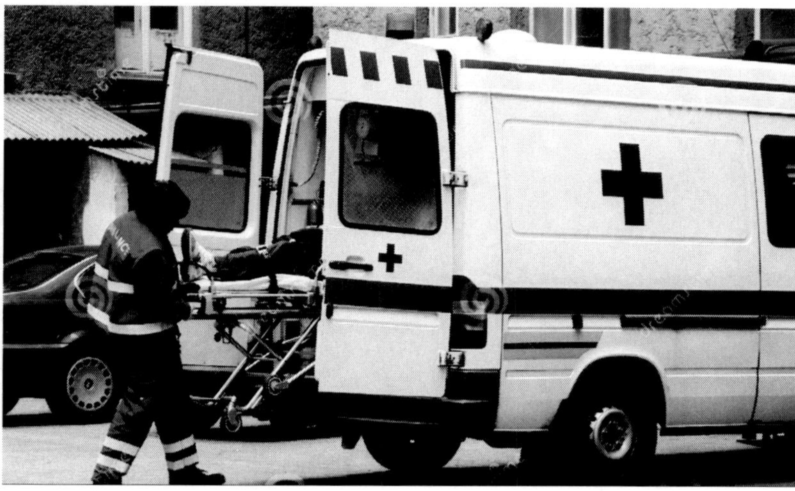

Unexpected problems can always arise. It helps to have a local physician or school clinic where they know you and can treat emergencies and help you navigate the local medical system if specialized care is necessary.

Safety

In the college years, most students are healthy and have few chronic disease issues. However, accidents are a leading cause of health issues. The most common accidents in college age men and women are the following:

- *Crosswalk injuries to pedestrians*
- *Bicycle injuries*
- *Slip and fall injuries*
- *Smoke inhalation and/or burns from fires started by hot plates*
- *Chemical burns from lab experiments*
- *Sports-related injuries*
- *Car crash injuries*

Mindfulness and Accident Prevention

There are many accident prevention guidelines, pamphlets and recommendations to decrease accidents in general, but that is not the purpose of this book. However, I do want to stress that many, if not most accidents and injuries in college could be prevented with mindfulness.

The other day I drove from my house early in the morning to work. I was thinking about my coming day and realized when I arrived at work that I was completely unaware of driving to work. I did not remember one turn, one stop light…it was as if I was at home one minute and transported magically to work the next. Often when we are preoccupied or doing repetitive tasks with which we are very familiar, we go on autopilot. This is a recipe for accident disaster. Since that day I have vowed to remain mindful on the road.

The definition I like for mindfulness in the context of accident prevention is paying attention in a particular way: on purpose, in the present moment, without judgment. For college students to be mindful in the classroom, dorm, and on campus requires a personal commitment to stay in the present moment, stay focused, and be keenly aware of the environment. Strategies that stress healthy behaviors both physical and psychological, boost stamina, and allow for recharging and relaxation motivate students to stay mindful. But it is not just the individual student who must remain mindful: the school organization itself must set the example by adopting a policy of mindfulness. To promote organizational mindfulness on college campuses requires:

- Colleges to have systems in place for ease of reporting problems during office hours and after-hours and educating students on how to access those systems
- Commitment to safety
- Realistic and flexible norms and rules about dealing with and decreasing risk
- Colleges need to have the ability to reflect upon and improve practices through monitoring and analysis

All of us allow our minds to drift at times, and studies show that a "breather" every so often helps boost productivity. But many accidents happen even when accident prevention programs are in place and being followed. Mindfulness training on college campuses from the top of the organization down could potentially eliminate many school accidents.

The intention of this book has been to give you strategies to stay healthy in your life, both in college and at home. Taken together, the diet, lifestyle, safety and immune boosting, stress-reduction techniques outlined in these pages can significantly improve your health and possibly even save your life. It did mine. Keep it with you and leaf through if you have an issue that arises. It is my hope that the recommendations in this book will substantially benefit hard working college students.

Made in United States
North Haven, CT
24 September 2026

19102538R00035